THE HORMONE HARMONY COOKBOOK

A proven recipe for Healthy Cycles, PMS, PCOS to lose Weight, improve Fertility, Balance Hormone, Menopause, Boost Energy and Mood, Treat Inflammation and Fix Metabolism.

Olivia Jones

TABLE OF CONTENTS

INTRODUCTION

Introduction to Hormone Balancing Diet

Maintaining a proper hormonal balance is crucial for one's overall health and well-being. Hormones are instrumental in regulating a multitude of bodily functions, such as metabolism, mood, sleep, and reproductive health. However, factors like stress, poor diet, environmental toxins, and certain medical conditions can disrupt our hormonal equilibrium.

In the bustling city of Wellnessville, there lived a vibrant woman named Emma. Despite her energetic spirit, Emma found herself entangled in the complexities of hormone imbalance, a challenge that cast shadows over her daily life. Fatigue, mood swings, and persistent skin issues became unwelcome companions on her journey.

One day, as she navigated through the sea of health advice, Emma stumbled upon a transformative realization—her diet held the key to unlocking the elusive harmony her body craved. Inspired and determined, she embarked on a culinary adventure, exploring the intersection of flavor and hormonal equilibrium.

The " Harmony Within Cookbook: Balancing Your Body Naturally" is a collection of the recipes and wisdom that guided Emma back to vitality. Each dish became a chapter in her narrative of renewal, as nutrient-rich ingredients and mindful preparation became her allies in the quest for balance.

Join us on a journey through this cookbook, where the tale of Emma's triumph unfolds in recipes carefully crafted to nourish not just the body, but the soul. Discover the power of a well-balanced plate as we delve into the delicious world of Hormone Harmony—a culinary odyssey that promises not just meals, but a roadmap to radiant well-being.

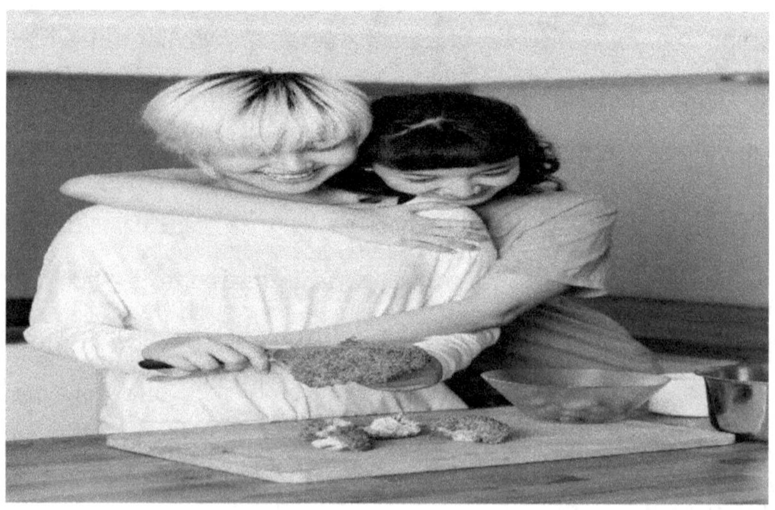

CHAPTER ONE

Breakfast Recipes

1.1 Hormone Balancing Smoothie Bowl

Ingredients:

1 banana

1 cup frozen mixed berries

1 tablespoon chia seeds

1 tablespoon flaxseed meal

1 cup unsweetened almond milk

Toppings of choice: sliced almonds, coconut flakes, fresh berries

Preparation:

- In a blender, combine the banana, frozen berries, chia seeds, flaxseed meal, and almond milk.
- Blend until smooth and creamy.
- Pour the smoothie into a bowl and enhance it with the toppings of your liking.

Benefits:

- This smoothie bowl is rich in antioxidants and fiber from the mixed berries, which can support hormone balance.
- Chia seeds and flaxseed meal are high in omega-3 fatty acids, which have anti-inflammatory properties and can aid in hormone regulation.
- Almonds provide healthy fats and protein, helping to stabilize blood sugar levels and promote satiety.

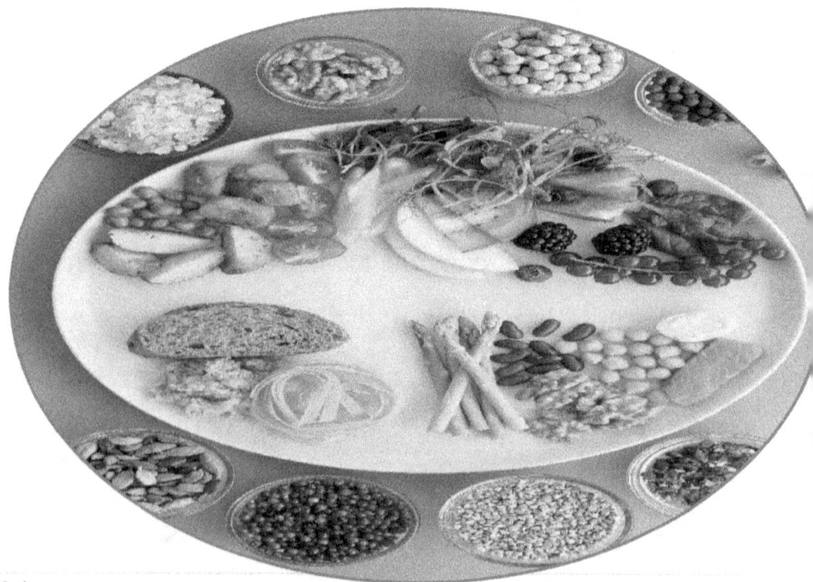

1.2 Flaxseed Pancakes with Berries

Ingredients:

1 cup oat flour

2 tablespoons ground flaxseed

1 teaspoon baking powder

1 tablespoon maple syrup

1 cup almond milk

Fresh berries for topping

Preparation:

- In a mixing bowl, combine oat flour, ground flaxseed, and baking powder.
- Add maple syrup and almond milk, stirring until well combined.
- Heat a non-stick pan over medium heat and lightly grease with cooking spray or coconut oil.
- Pour ¼ cup of batter onto the pan and cook until bubbles form on the surface. Flip and cook for another minute.

- Repeat with the remaining batter.

- Serve the pancakes with fresh berries on top.

Benefits:

- Flaxseed is rich in lignans, which have estrogen-like effects in the body and can support hormone balance.
- Oats provide complex carbohydrates and fiber, promoting sustained energy levels and supporting stable blood sugar levels.

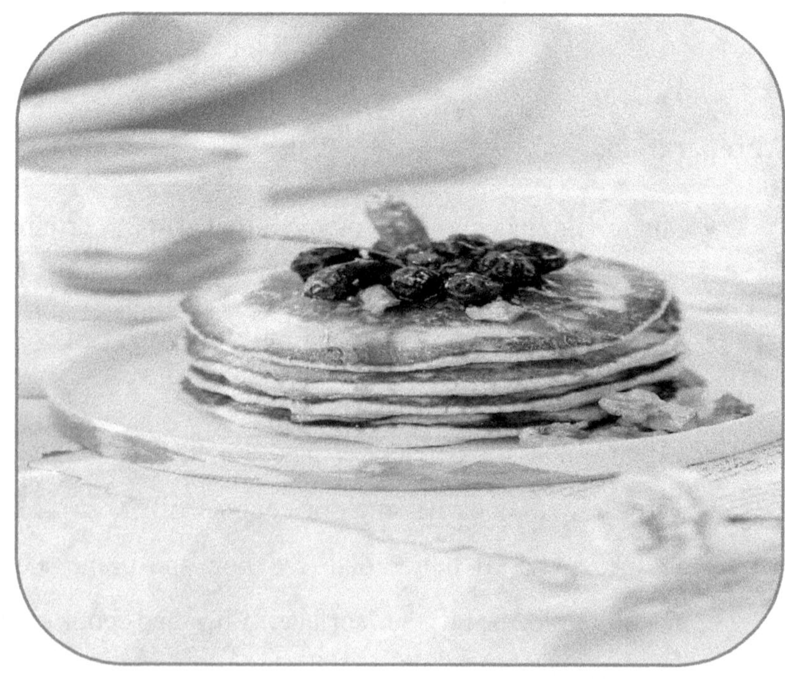

1.3 Avocado and Egg Toast

Ingredients:

2 slices whole grain bread

1 avocado, mashed

2 eggs

Salt and pepper to taste

Optional toppings: sliced tomatoes, sprouts, or microgreens

Preparation:

- Toast the slices of bread until they are perfectly golden brown.
- Spread mashed avocado evenly on each toast slice.
- In a non-stick skillet, cook the eggs to your preference (poached, fried, or scrambled).
- Arrange the boiled eggs on top of the avocado toast.
- Season with salt and pepper, and add any desired toppings.

Benefits:

- Avocado is rich in healthy monounsaturated fats, which are essential for hormone production and absorption.

- Eggs are a great source of protein, providing essential amino acids needed for hormone synthesis and regulation.

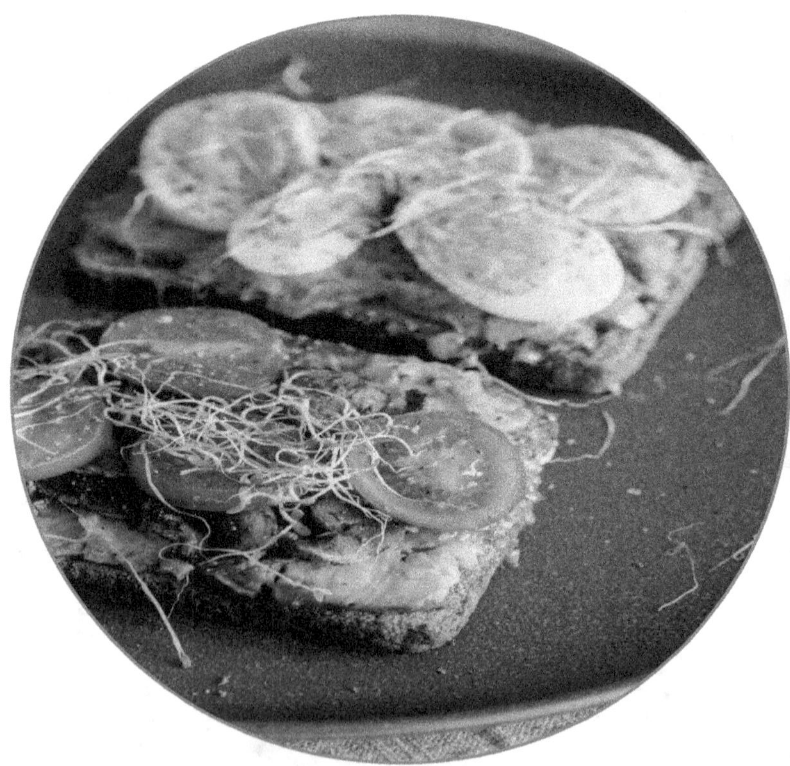

1.4 Quinoa Breakfast Bowl with Nuts and Seeds

Ingredients:

½ cup cooked quinoa

¼ cup Greek yogurt

1 tablespoon honey or maple syrup

1 tablespoon mixed nuts (almonds, walnuts, or cashews)

1 tablespoon mixed seeds (chia, pumpkin, or sunflower)

Fresh fruits for topping

Preparation:

- In a bowl, mix cooked quinoa, Greek yogurt, and honey/maple syrup until well combined.
- Top the quinoa mixture with mixed nuts, seeds, and fresh fruits.

Benefits:

- Quinoa is a plant-based source of complete protein and contains essential amino acids that aid in hormone balance.

- Greek yogurt provides probiotics, which can support gut health and indirectly influence hormone regulation.

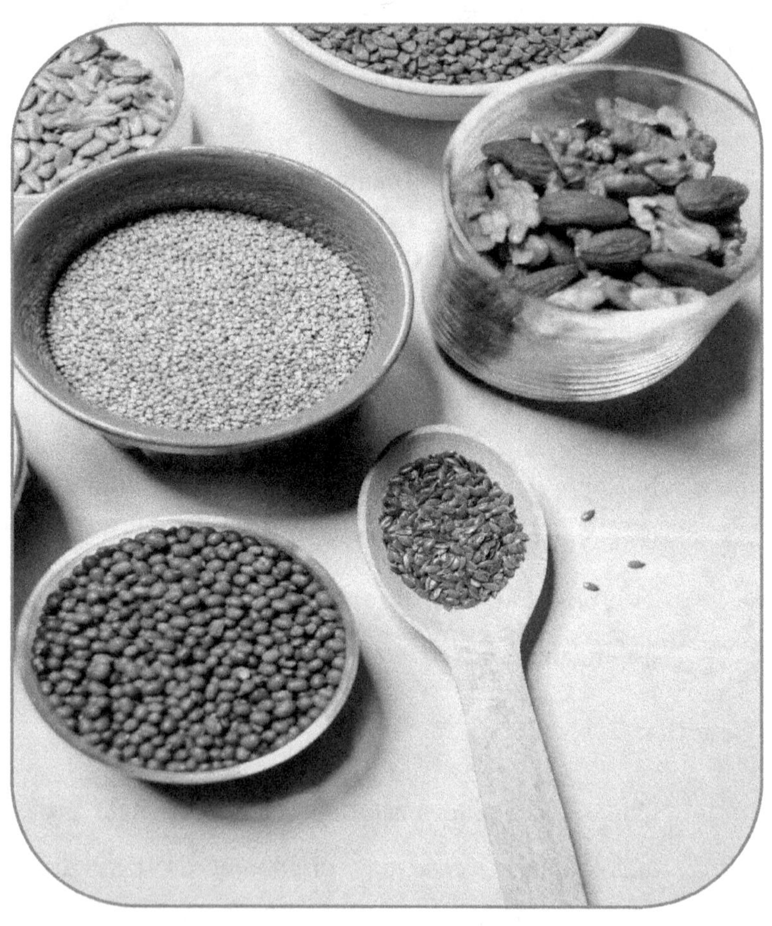

1.5 Chia Seed Pudding with Mixed Berries

Ingredients:

3 tablespoons chia seeds

1 cup unsweetened almond milk

1 tablespoon honey or maple syrup

½ teaspoon vanilla extract

Mixed berries for topping

Preparation:

- In a glass jar or bowl, mix chia seeds, almond milk, honey/maple syrup, and vanilla extract.
- Mix thoroughly to blend and make sure the chia seeds are evenly spread.
- Place the jar/bowl in the refrigerator and let it sit overnight or for at least a couple of hours.
- Before serving, stir the chia seed mixture to break up any clumps.
- Top with mixed berries.

Benefits:

- Chia seeds are packed with omega-3 fatty acids and fiber, which can aid in hormonal regulation and support digestive health.
- Almond milk provides a dairy-free option that is low in calories and can be easily digested.

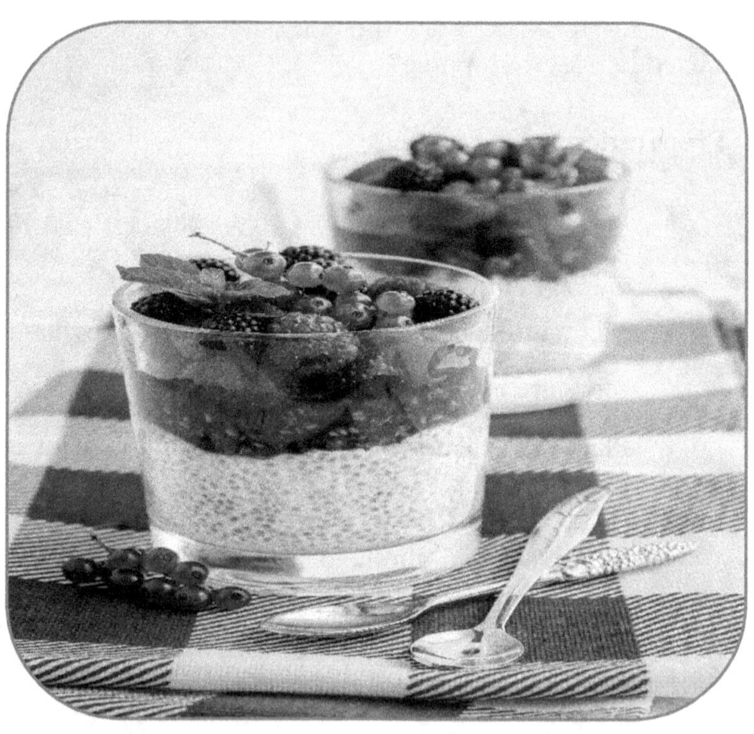

CHAPTER TWO

Lunch Recipes

2.1 Salmon and Quinoa Salad with Lemon Dressing

Ingredients:

4 oz grilled salmon fillet

1 cup cooked quinoa

2 cups mixed greens

1/2 cucumber, sliced

1/4 cup cherry tomatoes, halved

1/4 cup red onion, thinly sliced

2 tablespoons sliced almonds

For the Lemon Dressing:

2 tablespoons fresh lemon juice

2 tablespoons extra-virgin olive oil

1 teaspoon Dijon mustard

Salt and pepper to taste

Preparation:

- In a bowl, combine the cooked quinoa, mixed greens, cucumber, cherry tomatoes, red onion, and sliced almonds.
- In a separate small bowl, whisk together the lemon juice, olive oil, Dijon mustard, salt, and pepper to make the dressing.
- Pour the lemon dressing over the salad and mix it in.
- Top the salad with grilled salmon fillet.
- Serve and enjoy.

Benefits:

- Salmon is rich in omega-3 fatty acids, which can help reduce inflammation and support hormone balance.
- Quinoa is a high-protein grain substitute that provides essential amino acids and fiber for sustained energy and balanced blood sugar levels.
- Mixed greens and vegetables provide a variety of vitamins, minerals, and antioxidants to support overall health and hormonal function.

2.2 Hormone Balancing Buddha Bowl

Ingredients:

1 cup cooked brown rice

1 cup roasted sweet potatoes, cubed

1 cup steamed broccoli florets

1/2 cup cooked chickpeas

1/4 avocado, sliced

2 tablespoons tahini

2 tablespoons lemon juice

1 tablespoon tamari or soy sauce

1 tablespoon nutritional yeast (optional)

Salt and pepper to taste

Preparation:

- In a bowl, arrange the cooked brown rice, roasted sweet potatoes, steamed broccoli florets, cooked chickpeas, and sliced avocado.

- In a separate small bowl, whisk together the tahini, lemon juice, tamari or soy sauce, nutritional yeast (if using), salt, and pepper to make the dressing.
- Drizzle the dressing over the Buddha bowl.

Serve and enjoy.

Benefits:

- Brown rice is a complex carbohydrate that provides steady energy and essential nutrients without causing blood sugar spikes.
- Sweet potatoes are rich in fiber and vitamins A and C, which can support hormone production and immune function.
- Broccoli is a cruciferous vegetable that contains compounds known as indoles, which may help maintain hormonal balance.
- Chickpeas are a good source of plant-based protein and fiber, supporting overall health and hormone regulation.
- Avocado and tahini are healthy fats that provide essential fatty acids necessary for hormone synthesis.

2.3 Vegetable Stir-Fry with Tofu

Ingredients:

1 cup firm tofu, cubed

1 cup mixed vegetables (bell peppers, broccoli, snap peas, carrots, etc.)

2 cloves garlic, minced

1 tablespoon vegetable oil

1 tablespoon tamari or soy sauce

1 tablespoon sesame oil

1 teaspoon ginger, grated

Sesame seeds for garnish (optional)

Fresh cilantro for garnish (optional)

Preparation:

- In a skillet or wok, heat vegetable oil over medium-high heat.
- Add minced garlic and grated ginger, and stir for a minute until fragrant.
- Add tofu cubes and cook until lightly browned.

- Add mixed vegetables and tamari or soy sauce. stir-fry the vegetable for approximately 3-4 minutes until they reach a tender-crisp texture.

- Sprinkle with sesame oil and toss everything together.

- Garnish with sesame seeds and fresh cilantro (if desired).

- Serve the stir-fry alone or over cooked quinoa or brown rice.

Benefits:

- Tofu is a plant-based protein source that can be beneficial for hormone balance, as it contains isoflavones that have estrogen-like effects in the body.

- Mixed vegetables provide a variety of vitamins, minerals, and fiber that support overall health and hormonal function.

- Garlic and ginger have anti-inflammatory properties and may help in reducing inflammation and balancing hormones.

- Sesame oil adds a nutty flavor and contains healthy fats that support hormone production and absorption.

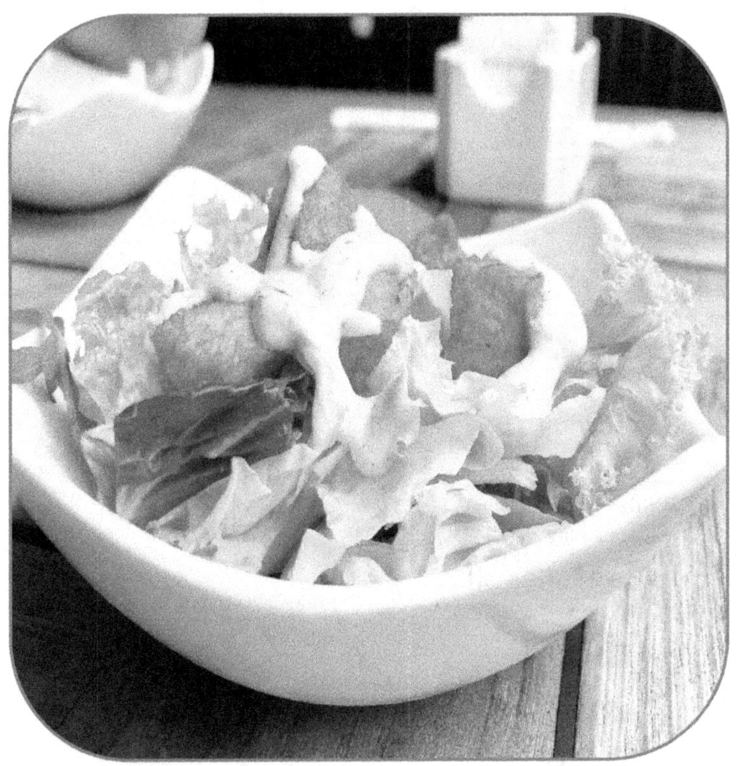

2.4 Chickpea Salad with Avocado Dressing

Ingredients:

1 can chickpeas, drained and rinsed

1 cup cherry tomatoes, halved

1 cucumber, diced

1/4 cup red onion, thinly sliced

2 tablespoons fresh parsley, chopped

For the Avocado Dressing:

1 ripe avocado

2 tablespoons lemon juice

1 tablespoon olive oil

1 clove garlic, minced

Salt and pepper to taste

Preparation:

- In a large bowl, combine chickpeas, cherry tomatoes, cucumber, red onion, and chopped parsley.

- In a separate bowl, mash the ripe avocado with a fork until smooth.

- Add lemon juice, olive oil, minced garlic, salt, and pepper to the mashed avocado and stir until well combined to make the dressing.

- Pour the avocado dressing over the chickpea salad and toss to coat evenly.

The salad can be enjoyed either chilled or at room temperature.

Benefits:

- Chickpeas are a good source of plant-based protein and fiber, helping to regulate blood sugar levels and support hormone balance.

- Cherry tomatoes and cucumber provide hydration, antioxidants, and nutrients to support overall health and hormonal function.

- Avocado is rich in healthy monounsaturated fats, which are essential for hormone production and absorption.

- Fresh parsley adds flavor and is known for its potential to support detoxification and hormone regulation.

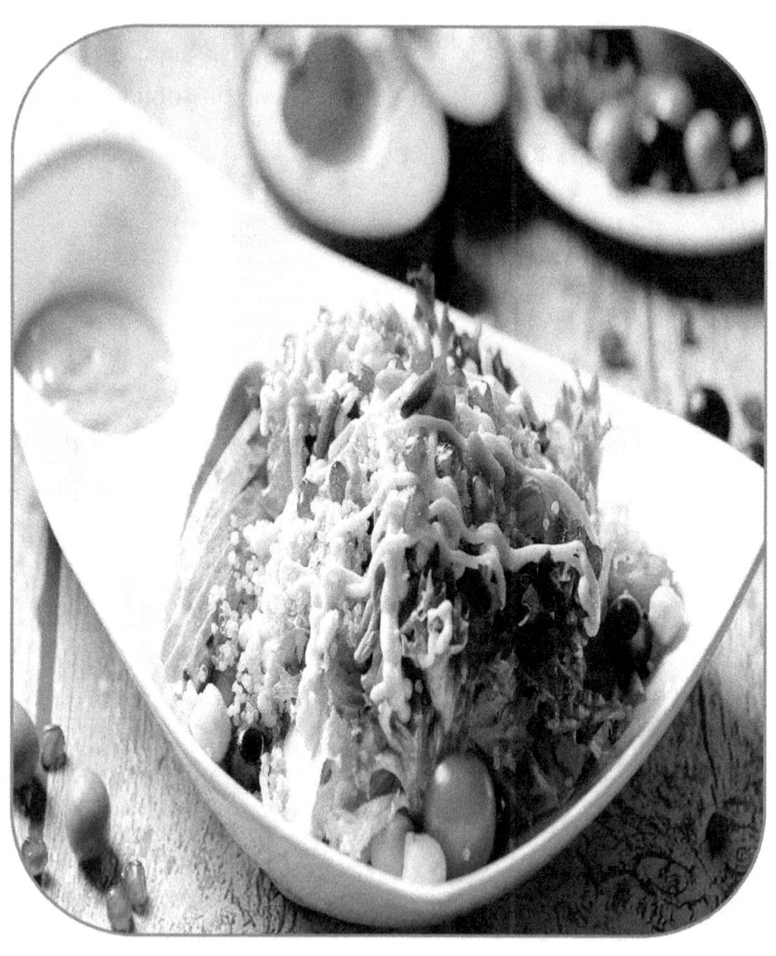

2.5 Mediterranean Quinoa Salad

Ingredients:

1 cup cooked quinoa

1/2 cup canned chickpeas, drained and rinsed

1/2 cup Kalamata olives, pitted and halved

1/2 cup cherry tomatoes, halved

1/4 cup red onion, thinly sliced

1/4 cup crumbled feta cheese (optional)

2 tablespoons fresh parsley, chopped

For the Dressing:

2 tablespoons lemon juice

2 tablespoons extra-virgin olive oil

1 clove garlic, minced

1 teaspoon dried oregano

Salt and pepper to taste

Preparation:

- In a large bowl, combine cooked quinoa, chickpeas, Kalamata olives, cherry tomatoes, red onion, crumbled feta cheese (if using), and chopped parsley.
- In a small bowl, whisk together lemon juice, olive oil, minced garlic, dried oregano, salt, and pepper to make the dressing.
- Combine the quinoa salad with the dressing by drizzling it over and tossing gently.

The salad can be served either chilled or at room temperature.

Benefits:

- Quinoa is a nutrient-dense grain substitute that provides essential amino acids and fiber for sustained energy and balanced blood sugar levels.
- Chickpeas offer a good source of plant-based protein and fiber, aiding in hormone balance and satiety.
- Kalamata olives contain healthy monounsaturated fats and antioxidants that support cardiovascular health and hormone production.

- Fresh parsley adds flavor and potential hormone-balancing properties due to its high vitamin C and antioxidants content.

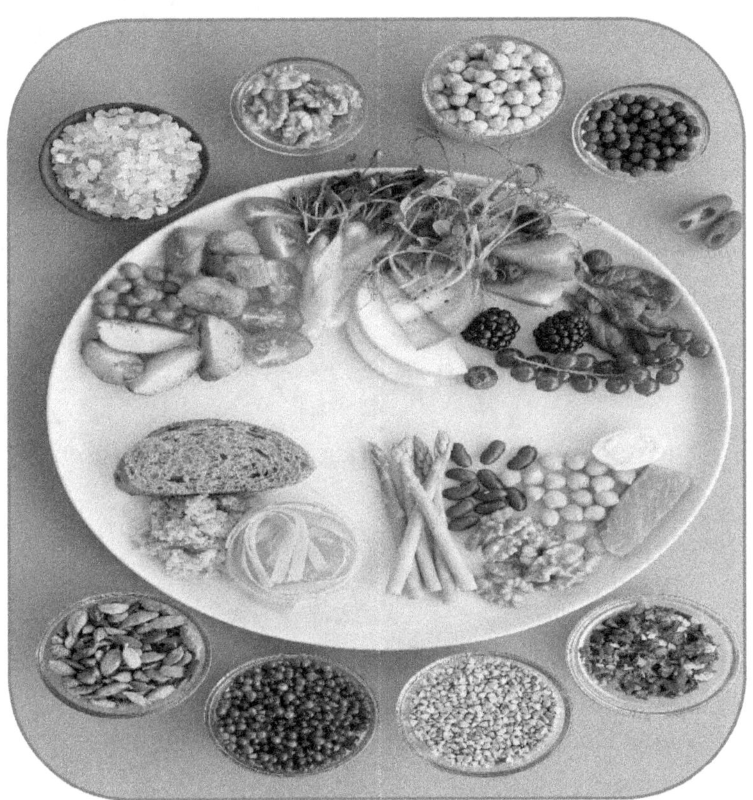

CHAPTER THREE

Dinner Recipes

3.1 Grilled Chicken with Roasted Vegetables

Ingredients:

4 oz chicken breast

1 cup mixed vegetables (broccoli, bell peppers, zucchini, carrots)

1 tablespoon olive oil

1 teaspoon dried herbs (such as thyme, rosemary, or oregano)

Salt and pepper to taste

Preparation:

- Heat the grill or grill pan to medium-high.
- Season the chicken breast with dried herbs, salt, and pepper.
- Drizzle olive oil over the mixed vegetables and season with salt and pepper.

- Grill the chicken for about 6-8 minutes per side until cooked through.
- At the same time, roast the mixed vegetables in the oven at 400°F for 15-20 minutes until tender.

Serve the grilled chicken with a side of roasted vegetables.

Benefits:

- Chicken breast is a lean protein source that provides essential amino acids for hormone synthesis and muscle repair.
- Mixed vegetables offer an array of vitamins, minerals, and antioxidants for overall health and hormonal balance.
- Olive oil provides healthy monounsaturated fats, which are beneficial for hormone production and absorption.

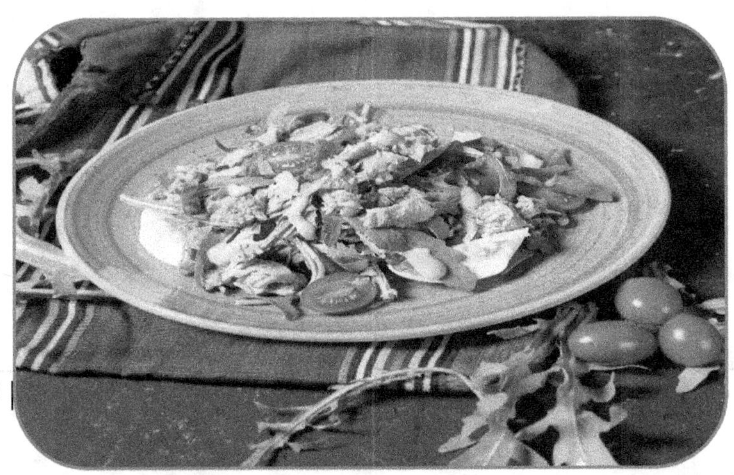

3.2 Baked Salmon with Steamed Asparagus

Ingredients:

4 oz salmon fillet

1 bunch asparagus

1 tablespoon olive oil

1 garlic clove, minced

Juice of 1/2 lemon

Salt and pepper to taste

Preparation:

- Preheat the oven to 400°F.
- Line a baking sheet with parchment paper and place the salmon fillet on top.
- Drizzle olive oil over the salmon and season with minced garlic, lemon juice, salt, and pepper.
- Bake the salmon for about 12-15 minutes until cooked through and flaky.
- Meanwhile, steam the asparagus until tender, about 3-5 minutes.

Serve the baked salmon with steamed asparagus on the side.

Benefits:

- Salmon is rich in omega-3 fatty acids, which can help reduce inflammation and support hormone balance.

- Asparagus is a nutrient-dense vegetable that provides fiber, folate, and other essential nutrients that may promote hormonal regulation and overall health.

- Olive oil adds healthy monounsaturated fats and enhances the flavor of the dish.

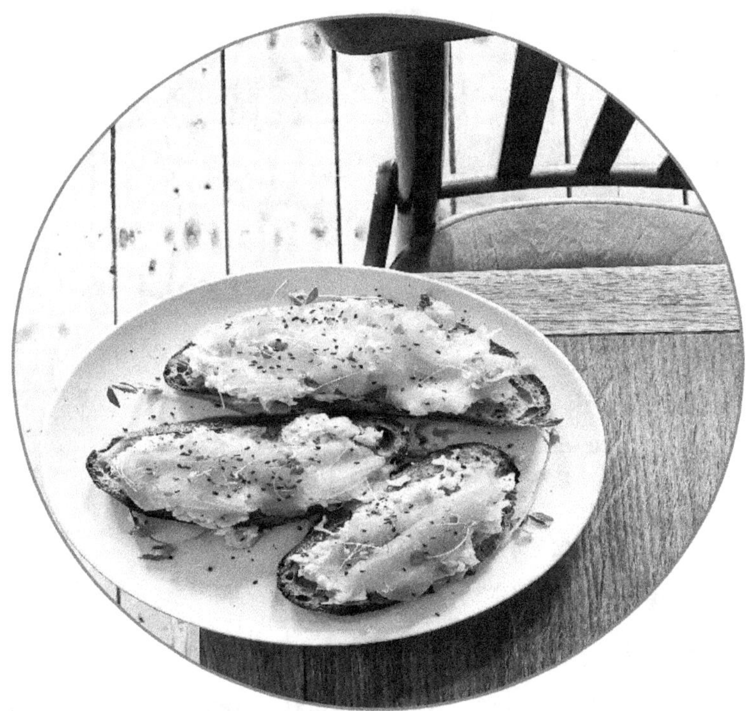

3.3 Quinoa Stuffed Bell Peppers

Ingredients:

2 large bell peppers (any color)

1 cup cooked quinoa

1/2 cup black beans, rinsed and drained

1/2 cup corn kernels

1/2 cup diced tomatoes

1/4 cup red onion, finely chopped

1/4 cup shredded cheddar cheese or dairy-free alternative

1 tablespoon chopped fresh cilantro

1 teaspoon cumin

Salt and pepper to taste

Preparation:

- Preheat the oven to 400°F.
- Remove the tops of the bell peppers and discard the seeds and membranes.
- In a mixing bowl, combine cooked quinoa, black beans, corn kernels, diced tomatoes, red onion,

shredded cheese, chopped cilantro, cumin, salt, and pepper.

- Fill the bell peppers with the quinoa mixture and arrange them in a baking dish.
- Cover the baking dish with foil and bake for 25-30 minutes until the bell peppers are tender.
- Take off the foil and continue baking for 5 more minutes until the cheese is melted.

Serve the quinoa stuffed bell peppers hot.

Benefits:

- Quinoa is a complete protein source that contains essential amino acids needed for hormone synthesis and regulation.
- Bell peppers are rich in vitamins A and C, which are important for hormonal health and immune function.
- Black beans provide fiber and plant-based protein, promoting satiety and supporting hormone balance.
- Cumin adds flavor and may have potential anti-inflammatory properties.

3.4 Lentil Curry with Cauliflower Rice

Ingredients:

1 cup red lentils

1 small onion, chopped

2 cloves garlic, minced

1 tablespoon curry powder

1 teaspoon turmeric

1/2 teaspoon cumin

1/2 teaspoon paprika

1 can coconut milk

2 cups cauliflower rice

Fresh cilantro for garnish (optional)

Salt and pepper to taste

Preparation:

- Rinse the red lentils thoroughly.
- In a large saucepan, sauté the chopped onion and minced garlic until fragrant.

- Add curry powder, turmeric, cumin, and paprika to the saucepan and stir for a minute to release the flavors.

- Add the red lentils and coconut milk to the saucepan. Bring to a boil, then reduce heat and simmer for about 15-20 minutes until the lentils are cooked and the mixture thickens.

- In a separate pan, sauté the cauliflower rice with a little olive oil until heated through.

- Season the lentil curry with salt and pepper to taste.

- Serve the lentil curry over cauliflower rice.

- Garnish with fresh cilantro if desired.

Benefits:

- Lentils are a plant-based source of protein, fiber, and essential nutrients that may support hormone balance and overall health.

- Cauliflower rice is a low-calorie, grain-free alternative that provides essential vitamins and minerals.

- Curry spices like turmeric and cumin have anti-inflammatory properties and may support healthy hormone production and regulation.

- Coconut milk adds a creamy texture and provides healthy fats that aid in hormone production and absorption.

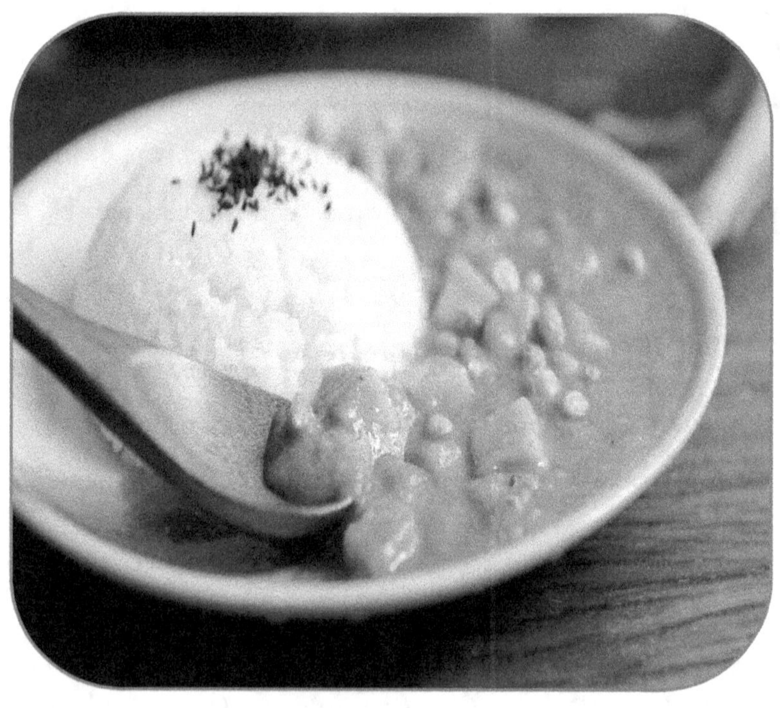

3.5 Zucchini Noodles with Pesto and Cherry Tomatoes

Ingredients:

4 oz chicken breast

1 cup Brussels sprouts, halved

1 tablespoon olive oil

1 garlic clove, minced

1/2 teaspoon dried thyme

Salt and pepper to taste

Preparation:

- Preheat the oven to 400°F.
- Season the chicken breast with salt, pepper, and dried thyme.
- In a mixing bowl, toss the halved Brussels sprouts with olive oil, minced garlic, salt, and pepper.

- Place the seasoned chicken breast and Brussels sprouts on a baking sheet lined with parchment paper.

- Bake for about 20-25 minutes until the chicken is cooked through and the Brussels sprouts are crispy and golden.

- Serve the baked chicken with roasted Brussels sprouts.

Benefits:

- Chicken breast is a lean protein source that provides essential amino acids for hormone synthesis and muscle repair.

- Brussels sprouts are loaded with vitamins, minerals, and antioxidants that contribute to hormonal balance and overall well-being.

- Olive oil adds healthy monounsaturated fats, which support hormone production and absorption.

- Garlic and thyme have potential anti-inflammatory properties and may help regulate hormones.

CHAPTER FOUR

Snack Recipes

4.1 Blueberry Chia Pudding

Ingredients:

1/4 cup chia seeds

1 cup unsweetened almond milk

1/2 cup blueberries

1 tablespoon honey or maple syrup (optional for sweetness)

1 tablespoon almond slices or shredded coconut for topping (optional)

Preparation:

- In a jar or bowl, mix the chia seeds and almond milk together.
- Stir well to avoid clumps, then let it sit for about 5 minutes.
- Stir the combination once more to break apart any clumps.

- Refrigerate and cover for a minimum of 2 hours or overnight to allow the chia seeds to soak up the liquid.

- Once the chia pudding has thickened to your desired consistency, stir in the blueberries and sweeten with honey or maple syrup if desired.

- Divide the pudding into serving bowls or jars and top with almond slices or shredded coconut, if desired.

Serve chilled.

Benefits:

- Chia seeds are rich in omega-3 fatty acids and fiber, supporting hormonal balance and digestion.

- Blueberries are packed with antioxidants that help reduce inflammation and protect against cellular damage.

- Almond milk provides a dairy-free alternative and contains vitamin E, which plays a role in hormone regulation.

- Honey or maple syrup can add natural sweetness without causing sharp blood sugar spikes.

4.2 Kale Chips

Ingredients:

1 bunch kale, stems removed and torn into bite-sized pieces

1 tablespoon olive oil

1/2 teaspoon garlic powder

1/2 teaspoon paprika

Salt to taste

Preparation:

- Preheat the oven to 350°F.
- Place the torn kale pieces in a large bowl.
- Drizzle olive oil over the kale and sprinkle with garlic powder, paprika, and salt.
- Massage the oil and seasonings into the kale leaves until they are evenly coated.
- Arrange the kale in a single layer on a baking sheet that is lined with parchment paper.
- Bake for 10-15 minutes until the kale becomes crispy but not burnt.
- Allow the kale chips to cool before serving.

Benefits:

- Kale is a nutrient-dense leafy green vegetable that contains high amounts of vitamins A, C, and K, which are important for hormone synthesis and immune function.

- Olive oil provides healthy monounsaturated fats that support hormone production and absorption.

- Garlic powder adds flavor and potentially has antibacterial and anti-inflammatory properties.

- Paprika contains antioxidants that may help regulate hormone levels and reduce oxidative stress.

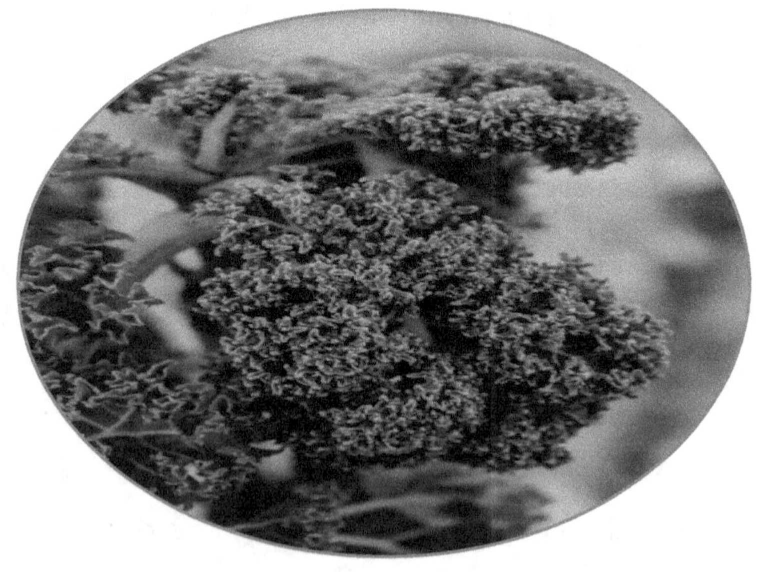

4.3 Energy Bites

Ingredients:

1 cup rolled oats

1/2 cup almond butter or any nut butter of your choice

1/4 cup honey or maple syrup

1/4 cup unsweetened shredded coconut

1/4 cup dark chocolate chips

2 tablespoons chia seeds

1 teaspoon vanilla extract

Pinch of salt

Preparation:

- Combine all the ingredients in a large bowl until thoroughly mixed.
- Cover and refrigerate the mixture for about 30 minutes to allow it to firm up.
- Once the mixture has chilled, roll it into small balls using your hands.

- Position the energy bites on a baking sheet that is lined with parchment paper.
- Refrigerate for at least 1 hour to set.

Keep the energy bites in an airtight container in the refrigerator until you are ready to enjoy them.

Benefits:

- Oats are a great source of fiber, which helps regulate blood sugar levels and supports overall hormonal function.
- Almond butter provides healthy fats and proteins that contribute to hormone synthesis and satiety.
- Honey or maple syrup adds natural sweetness without causing a significant spike in blood sugar levels.
- Shredded coconut and chia seeds offer additional fiber, micronutrients, and omega-3 fatty acids that promote hormonal balance and overall well-being.
- Dark chocolate chips, when consumed in moderate amounts, provide antioxidants and can help boost mood and energy levels.

4.4 Greek Yogurt Parfait

Ingredients:

1 cup Greek yogurt

1/2 cup mixed berries (strawberries, blueberries, raspberries)

1/4 cup granola

1 tablespoon honey or maple syrup (optional for sweetness)

Preparation:

- Layer the Greek yogurt, mixed berries, and granola in a glass or bowl.
- Repeat the layering process until all the ingredients have been used.
- Drizzle honey or maple syrup over the parfait for added sweetness if desired.
- Serve immediately.

Benefits:

- Greek yogurt is high in protein and low in sugar, making it a nutritious choice that supports muscle repair and hormone synthesis.

- Mixed berries are rich in antioxidants, vitamins, and minerals that promote overall well-being and hormonal balance.

- Granola provides fiber and healthy carbohydrates, giving you sustained energy and supporting healthy digestion.

- Honey or maple syrup can add natural sweetness without causing sharp blood sugar spikes.

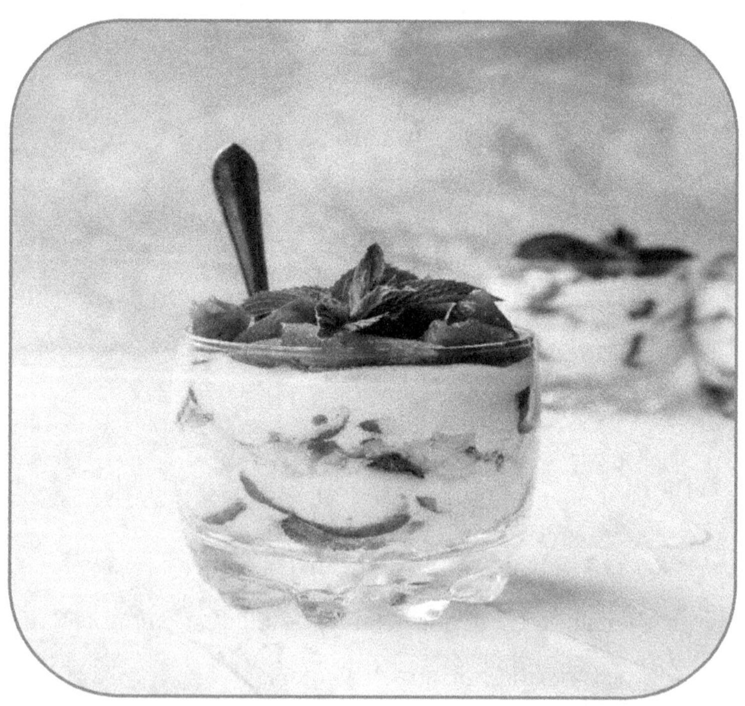

4.5 Avocado Toast

Ingredients:

2 slices whole grain bread

1 ripe avocado

1 tablespoon lemon juice

1/4 teaspoon red pepper flakes (optional)

Salt and pepper to taste

Optional toppings: sliced tomato, sliced radishes, microgreens

Preparation:

- Toast the slices of whole grain bread to your desired level of crispness.
- In a bowl, mash the ripe avocado with lemon juice, red pepper flakes (if using), salt, and pepper.
- Spread the mashed avocado mixture evenly onto the toasted bread slices.
- Top with optional toppings like sliced tomato, sliced radishes, or microgreens.
- If desired, sprinkle with additional salt and pepper.

Serve immediately.

Benefits:

- Whole grain bread provides complex carbohydrates and dietary fiber, promoting balanced blood sugar levels and aiding digestion.
- Avocado is rich in healthy monounsaturated fats that contribute to hormonal health and satiety.
- Lemon juice adds a refreshing taste and provides vitamin C, which is important for collagen synthesis and hormone production.
- Red pepper flakes can boost metabolism and provide a slight kick of heat.
- Optional toppings like tomatoes, radishes, and microgreens add extra nutrients, color, and flavor to the dish.

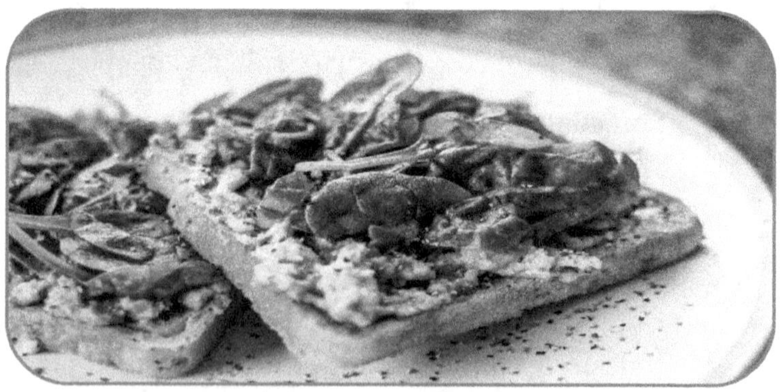

CHAPTER FIVE

Bonus Recipes

5.1 Cucumber and Hummus Bites

Ingredients:

1 large cucumber, sliced

1/2 cup hummus

Cherry tomatoes, sliced (optional for garnish)

Fresh herbs (such as parsley or dill), chopped (optional for garnish)

Preparation:

Slice the cucumber into rounds of about 1/4 inch thickness.

Spoon a small dollop of hummus onto each cucumber slice.

If desired, garnish with a slice of cherry tomato and/or sprinkle with fresh herbs.

Serve immediately.

Benefits:

- Cucumbers are hydrating and low in calories, providing a refreshing snack that supports hydration and overall well-being.

- Hummus is made with chickpeas, which are rich in fiber and plant-based protein, promoting satiety and aiding in hormone balance.

- Cherry tomatoes add a burst of flavor and provide antioxidants like lycopene, which may have anti-inflammatory properties.

- Fresh herbs not only enhance the taste but also offer additional vitamins and minerals.

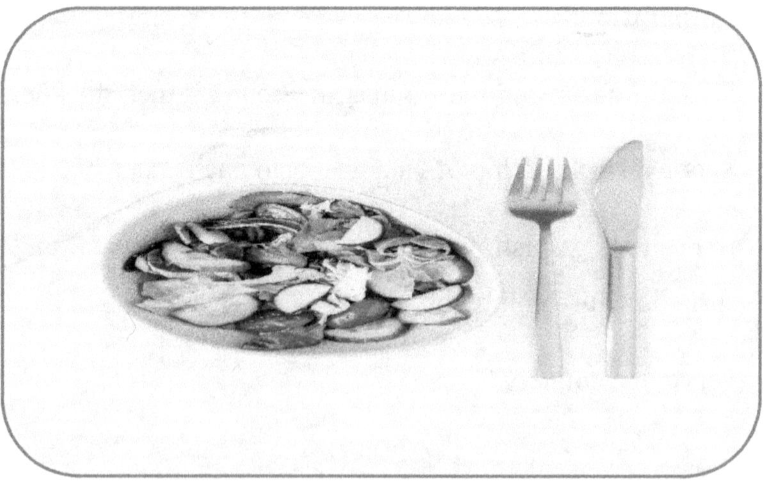

5.2 Almond Butter Energy Balls

Ingredients:

1 cup rolled oats

1/2 cup almond butter

1/4 cup honey or maple syrup

1/4 cup ground flaxseeds

1/4 cup dark chocolate chips

1 teaspoon vanilla extract

Pinch of salt

Preparation:

- In a large bowl, mix together all the ingredients until well combined.
- Cover and refrigerate the mixture for about 30 minutes to allow it to firm up.
- Once chilled, roll the mixture into bite-sized balls using your hands.
- Place the energy balls on a tray lined with parchment paper.
- Refrigerate for at least 1 hour to set.

- Store the energy balls in an airtight container in the refrigerator until ready to enjoy.

Benefits:

- Rolled oats provide fiber and slow-releasing carbohydrates, giving you sustained energy and supporting healthy digestion.

- Almond butter offers a good source of healthy fats, protein, and vitamin E, which are essential for hormone synthesis and overall well-being.

- Honey or maple syrup adds natural sweetness without causing sharp blood sugar spikes.

- Ground flaxseeds are rich in omega-3 fatty acids, fiber, and lignans, which can help balance hormones and support cardiovascular health.

- Dark chocolate chips, in moderation, provide antioxidants and can help boost mood and energy levels.

5.3 Veggie sticks with Greek Yogurt Dip

Ingredients:

Assorted vegetable sticks (carrots, celery, bell peppers, cucumber)

1 cup Greek yogurt

1 tablespoon lemon juice

1/2 teaspoon dried dill

1/4 teaspoon garlic powder

Salt and pepper to taste

Preparation:

- Wash and cut the vegetables into sticks.
- In a bowl, mix together the Greek yogurt, lemon juice, dried dill, garlic powder, salt, and pepper until well combined.
- Transfer the dip to a serving bowl.
- Arrange the vegetable sticks on a platter or plate alongside the Greek yogurt dip.

Serve immediately.

- Vegetable sticks are packed with vitamins, minerals, and fiber that support hormonal balance and overall health.

- Greek yogurt provides protein, calcium, and probiotics, which promote gut health and aid in hormone regulation.

- Lemon juice adds a tangy flavor and provides vitamin C, which is crucial for collagen synthesis and hormone production.

- Dried dill and garlic powder add a savory taste and potential anti-inflammatory benefits.

- This snack is low in calories and high in nutrients, making it a healthy option for hormone balancing and weight management.

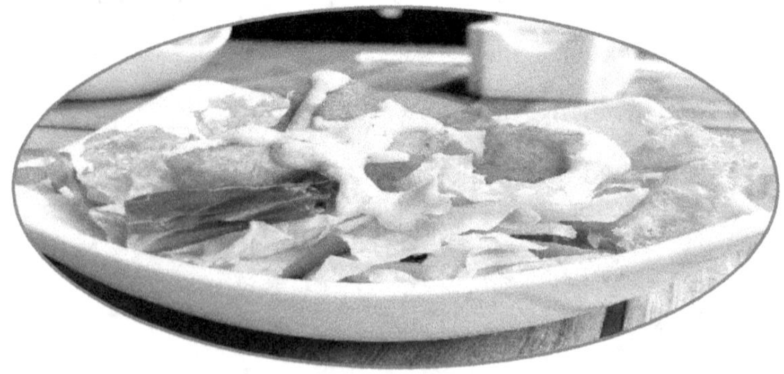

5.4 Berry Smoothie

Ingredients:

1 cup mixed berries (blueberries, strawberries, raspberries)

1 ripe banana

1 cup unsweetened almond milk or any milk of your choice

1 tablespoon honey or maple syrup (optional for sweetness)

Ice cubes (optional, for a chilled smoothie)

Preparation:

- Place the mixed berries, ripe banana, almond milk, and sweetener (if using) in a blender.
- Blend until smooth and creamy.
- If desired, add a few ice cubes and blend again until well combined and chilled.
- Pour the berry smoothie into a glass and serve immediately.

Benefits:

- Berries are rich in antioxidants, vitamins, and minerals that support hormonal balance, boost immune function, and protect against cellular damage.

- Ripe bananas provide natural sweetness and add texture to the smoothie. They are also a good source of potassium, which supports heart health and may help regulate blood pressure.

- Almond milk serves as a dairy-free base and adds a creamy texture. It is low in calories and contains vitamin E, which is important for hormonal health.

- Honey or maple syrup can be added for extra sweetness, although the natural sugars in the berries and banana should provide sufficient sweetness for most individuals.

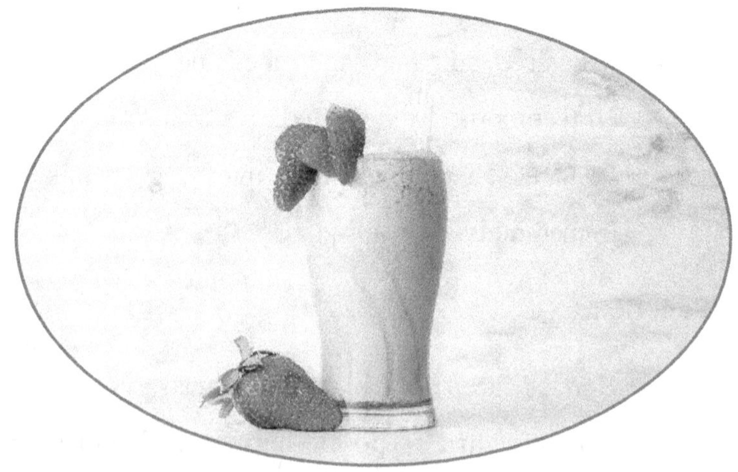

5.5 Quinoa Salad

Ingredients:

1 cup cooked quinoa

1 cup mixed vegetables (cucumber, cherry tomatoes, red onion cucumber, bell peppers)

1/4 cup crumbled feta cheese (optional)

2 tablespoons olive oil

1 tablespoon lemon juice

1 tablespoon chopped fresh herbs (such as basil or parsley)

Salt and pepper to taste

Preparation:

- In a large bowl, combine the cooked quinoa and mixed vegetables.
- If using, sprinkle in the crumbled feta cheese.
- Drizzle the olive oil and lemon juice over the salad mixture.
- Add the fresh herbs and season with salt and pepper.
- Toss the ingredients together until well combined.

Serve the quinoa salad chilled or at room temperature.

Benefits:

- Quinoa is a complete protein and a good source of fiber, aiding in hormonal balance, digestion, and satiety.
- Mixed vegetables provide a variety of vitamins, minerals, and antioxidants that support hormonal health and overall well-being.
- Feta cheese, in moderation, adds a tangy flavor and contributes protein and calcium to the salad.
- Olive oil offers heart-healthy monounsaturated fats and anti-inflammatory properties.
- Lemon juice acts as a natural flavor enhancer and provides vitamin C, which is important for hormone production and immune function.
- Fresh herbs not only add a burst of flavor but also contain beneficial compounds that may support hormonal balance and have antioxidant properties.

CHAPTER SIX

Tips for Hormone Balance

Tips for Maintaining a Hormone Balancing Diet

Plan your meals: Take the time to plan your meals and snacks in advance to ensure you have a variety of hormone-balancing options available throughout the week. By following this, you can maintain your focus and steer clear of making unhealthy food choices.

Prioritize whole foods: As much as possible, focus on consuming whole, unprocessed foods. These foods tend to be higher in nutrients and lower in additives, making them more supportive of hormonal balance.

Balance your macronutrients: Include a source of lean protein, healthy fats, and complex carbohydrates with every meal to maintain steady blood sugar levels and support hormone production.

Incorporate fiber: Aim to include fiber-rich foods like fruits, vegetables, whole grains, and legumes to support healthy digestion and hormone balance.

Stay hydrated: Proper hydration is essential for overall health, including hormone balance. Ensure you consume a sufficient quantity of water throughout the day to promote proper hydration and enhance your overall state of well-being.

Be mindful of portion sizes: Pay attention to portion sizes to avoid overeating and ensure you are consuming a balanced meal that aligns with your dietary needs and goals.

Listen to your body: Everyone's hormone balance is unique, so pay attention to how certain foods make you feel. Consider working with a healthcare professional or registered dietitian to tailor your diet to your specific needs.

Remember, maintaining a hormone balancing diet is not about strict rules or deprivation but rather about nourishing your body with wholesome foods and making sustainable choices that support your overall well-being. By following the recipes and tips provided, you can embark on a journey towards better hormone balance and improved health.

Lifestyle Tips for Hormone Balance

Stress-Reducing Practices

Mindfulness Meditation: Incorporate mindfulness meditation into your daily routine. Spending a few minutes in quiet reflection can help reduce stress and promote a sense of calm.

Deep Breathing Exercises: Practice deep breathing exercises to activate the body's relaxation response. Experiment with taking deep breaths through your nose, holding them for a brief period, and then exhaling slowly through your mouth.

Nature Connection: Spend time in nature regularly. Whether it's a walk in the park or simply sitting in a green space, connecting with nature can have a soothing effect on your nervous system.

Creative Outlets: Engage in creative activities that bring you joy, whether it's painting, writing, or playing music.

Expressing yourself creatively can be a therapeutic way to alleviate stress.

Exercise and Hormone Health

Regular Physical Activity: Incorporate regular exercise into your routine. Whether it's brisk walking, jogging, yoga, or weight training, physical activity promotes the release of endorphins and helps balance hormones.

Interval Training: Consider incorporating interval training into your workouts. Short bursts of intense exercise followed by rest periods have been shown to positively impact hormones like growth hormone and insulin.

Strength Training: Include strength training exercises in your fitness regimen. Building muscle mass can contribute to a healthy hormonal profile, especially in relation to insulin sensitivity.

Mind-Body Practices: Engage in mind-body practices such as yoga or tai chi to delve into the realm of harmonizing your mind and body. These activities not only provide physical benefits but also help regulate stress hormones and promote overall well-being.

Sleep Strategies for Balance

Consistent Sleep Schedule: Aim for a consistent sleep schedule by going to bed and waking up at the same time every day. By incorporating this practice, you can effectively regulate your body's internal rhythm.

Sleep Environment: Create a comfortable sleep environment. Keep your bedroom cool, dark, and quiet to optimize the conditions for restful sleep.

Digital Detox: Limit screen time before bedtime. The blue light emitted from screens can interfere with the production of the sleep hormone melatonin, making it harder to fall asleep.

Relaxation Techniques: Practice relaxation techniques before bedtime. This could include gentle stretching, reading a calming book, or practicing mindfulness to signal to your body that it's time to wind down.

Incorporating these lifestyle tips into your daily routine can contribute to hormonal balance and overall well-being. By adopting stress-reducing practices, staying physically active, and prioritizing restful sleep, you empower your body to function optimally and maintain hormonal harmony.

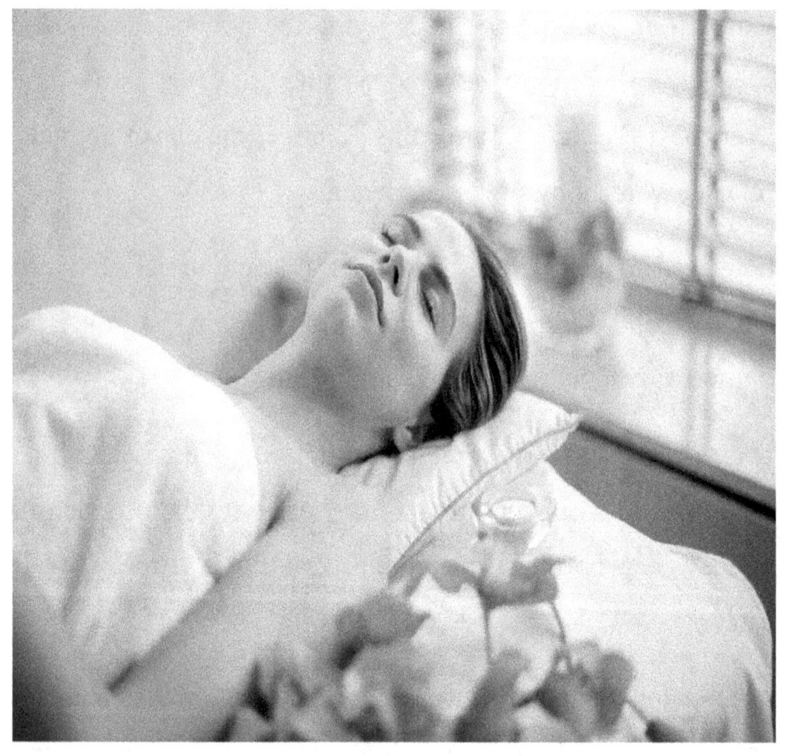

CHAPTER SEVEN

Conclusion

Your Journey to Hormone Harmony

As you embark on this culinary and lifestyle adventure towards hormonal balance, remember that it's not just about what you eat, but also how you live. The recipes shared in this cookbook are more than a collection of delicious dishes—they are a celebration of the profound connection between food and hormonal harmony.

By choosing nutrient-rich, hormone-friendly ingredients and savoring the flavors of these wholesome recipes, you are nourishing your body from within. The carefully curated chapters guide you through a culinary journey that supports hormonal balance, one meal at a time.

But the journey doesn't end with the recipes. It extends into your daily life through mindful practices and intentional choices. Embrace stress-reducing activities, find joy in movement, and prioritize restful sleep. These lifestyle elements are integral to maintaining the delicate dance of hormones within your body.

Remember, balance is not a destination but a continuous, evolving journey. It's about embracing a lifestyle that honors your body's needs and fosters overall well-being. Each choice you make contributes to the intricate symphony of hormones, working harmoniously to support your health and vitality.

So, savor every bite, relish each moment of mindfulness, and cherish the profound connection between your lifestyle and hormonal balance. Your journey to hormone harmony is a personal exploration—an investment in your well-being that pays dividends for a lifetime.

Bon appétit and here's to a life of balance, health, and joy!